High Risk Pregnancy

Causes and Management

Akmal El-Mazny

CONTENTS

Contents

Contents

INTRODUCTION

- Although pregnancy is considered a normal physiological event, yet it may be complicated by a disease or a disorder that affects the health or endangers the life of the mother or the fetus.

- Abnormalities that develop during pregnancy may be directly related to pregnancy (obstetric) or not (non-obstetric).

- Obstetric abnormalities, such as maternal characteristics and problems in previous pregnancies, may increase the risk of morbidity or mortality for the mother or the fetus.

- Non-obstetric (medical or surgical) disorders frequently complicate pregnancy, and management sometimes differs from that for non-pregnant patients.

- High risk pregnancies require close monitoring, and sometimes referral to a specialized center for antenatal care and delivery.

- This book provides a comprehensive review of high risk pregnancy, emphasizing its causes and management, which will be of immense value for obstetricians and allied health professionals.

OBSTETRIC HISTORY AND EXAMINATION

Obstetric History

- Present obstetric history:

• Calculate expected date of delivery (EDD = LMP + 9 months + 7 days)

• Calculate duration of pregnancy

• Symptoms of pregnancy

• Warning symptoms

• Investigations done during pregnancy

• Medications taken during pregnancy

- Past obstetric history:

• Previous abortions / viable pregnancies

• Mode of delivery

• Gestational age and sex

• Previous antenatal or postnatal complications

- Medical history:

• Hypertension

• Diabetes

• Cardiac disease

• Renal disease

• Infectious disease (e.g. Hepatitis B or C, HIV ...)

Obstetric Examination

- <u>General examination:</u>

• Vital signs

• Weight and height

• Stature and gait

• CVS: flow murmurs

• Breasts and nipples

- <u>Abdominal examination:</u>

• Fundal level

• Leopold maneuvers

• Auscultation of fetal heart sounds

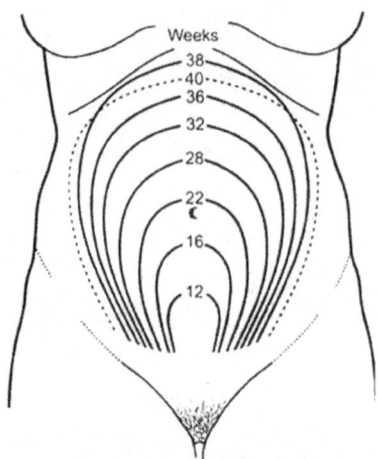

Fundal Level

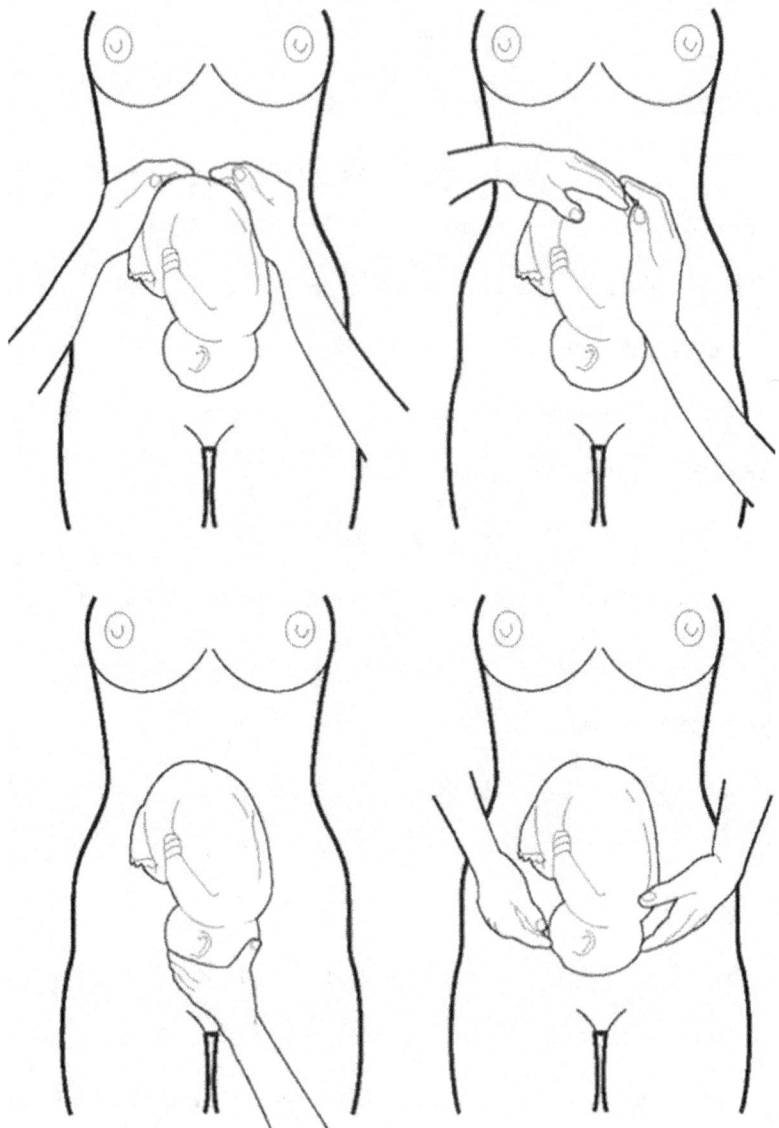

Leopold Maneuvers

ANTENATAL CARE

Objectives

- Prevention, early detection and treatment of pregnancy related complications as pre-eclampsia, eclampsia and hemorrhage

- Prevention, early detection and treatment of medical disorders as anemia and diabetes

- Detection of malpresentations, malpositions and disproportion that may influence the decision of labor

- Instructions about hygiene, diet and warning symptoms

- Laboratory studies of parameters may affect the fetus as blood group, Rh typing, toxoplasmosis and syphilis

Preconception Visit

- The ideal first visit should be at a preconception clinic where health education and risk assessment can be directed towards the planned pregnancy

- Advice can be given regarding the avoidance of harmful and teratogenic factors (drugs, cigarette smoking, alcohol intake …), ensuring an optimal dietary intake, and absence or control of chronic medical disorders (hypertension, diabetes …), in order to allow pregnancy to be started in the optimum conditions

Frequency of Antenatal Visits

- Every month during the first 6 months

- Every 2 weeks during the 7th and 8th months

- Every week during the last month

- More frequent visits are indicated in high risk pregnancy

The First Visit

- History: menstrual, obstetric, medical, surgical and family history

- Examination: general, abdominal and local

- Investigations:

• Blood grouping

• Rh typing

• Hemoglobin

• Urine analysis particularly for albumin and sugar

• Toxoplasma and VDRL if needed

Return Visits

- History: ask the patient about any complaint

- Examination:

• Weight

• Blood pressure

• Abdominal examination

• Edema

- <u>Investigations:</u>

• Urine for albumin and sugar

• Obstetric ultrasound if needed

- <u>Instructions:</u> about hygiene and diet

- <u>Warning symptoms:</u>

• Persistent headache

• Blurring of vision

• Persistent vomiting

• Abdominal pain

• Dimineshed fetal movements

• Vaginal bleaeding

• Gush of fluid per vagina

• Edema of lower limbs or face

ABORTION

Definition

- Loss of the pregnancy prior to viability (20 weeks or 500 gm)

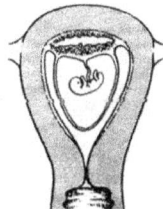 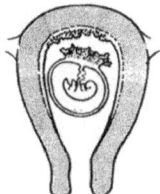 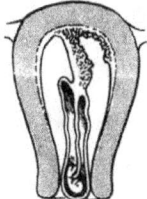 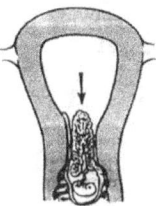

Types

- Threatened abortion

- Inevitable abortion

- Incomplete abortion

- Complete abortion

- Missed abortion

- Septic abortion

- Habitual abortion

- Therapeutic abortion

Causes

- Chromosomal abnormalities

- Infections (TORCHS ...)

- Immunological abnormalities

- Reproductive tract abnormalities (uterine abnormality, myoma, cervical incompetence ...)

- Endocrinal abnormalities (thyroid diseases, lutheal phase defect ...)

- Others (unknown, trauma, intoxication ...)

Diagnosis

- General:

• History of amenorrhea

• Vaginal bleeding

• Abdominal pain

• Endo-uterine bleeding on speculum

- Specific:

• Threatening abortion: the cervix is closed

• Inevitable abortion: the cervix is open and the products of conception are still in utero

• Incomplete abortion: the cervix is open and the products of conception are not com pletelyevacuated

• Complete abortion: the cervix is open and the products of conception are not present

• Missed abortion: the heart beat is absent

• Septic abortion: superimposed infection

• Habitual abortion: 3 or more successive spontaneous abortions

Complications

- Anemia

- Hypovolemic shock

- Septic shock

Investigations

- ß-HCG

- Obstetric ultrasound

- For repeated miscariage:

• Genetical investigations

• Infection screening

• Immunological profile

• Hysteroscopy

• Endocrine

Management

- Threatened abortion:

• Bed rest and review every week

• Progesterone

- Inevitable and incomplete abortion:

• Correct hypovolemic shock

• Surgical management: D & E (if uterus < 12 weeks)

• Medical management: Misoprostol (if uterus > 12 weeks)

- <u>Complete abortion:</u> reassure the patient

- <u>Missed abortion:</u>

• Surgical management: D & E (if uterus < 12 weeks)

• Medical management: Misoprostol (if uterus > 12 weeks)

- <u>Septic abortion:</u>

• Correct septic shock

• Surgical management: D & E (if uterus < 12 weeks)

• Medical management: Misoprostol (if uterus > 12 weeks)

• Antibiotics post-abortion

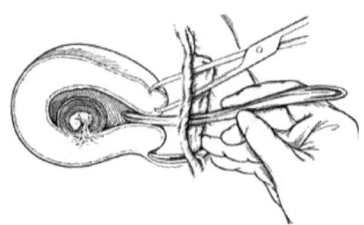 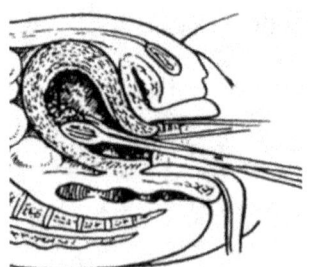

Surgical Evacuation (D & E)

CERVICAL INSUFFICIENCY

Definition

- Cervical dilation and shortening (anatomical or dysfunctional) leading to repetitive mid-tremister loss

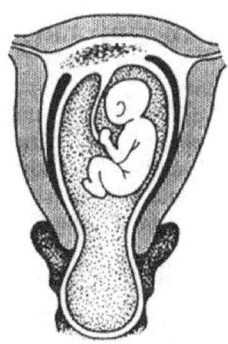

Causes

- Uterine anomalies (congenital cervical hypoplasia or aplasia ...)

- Prior cervical trauma (e.g. repeated D & C, other surgical procedures ...)

Diagnosis

- Recurrent mid trimester losses without contractions with a live fetus

- Premature rupture of membranes

Complications

- Habitual loss of the fetus

- Prematurity

- Premature rupture of membranes

Investigations

- Transvaginal ultrasound (cervical length < 25 mm, cervical dilatation, and funneling of membranes)

Management

- <u>Cerclage:</u> between 12 and 14 weeks of gestation

• Vaginal (McDonald's or Shirodkar)

• Abdominal

- <u>Decerclage:</u> at 37 weeks / contractions or CS (abdominal cerclage)

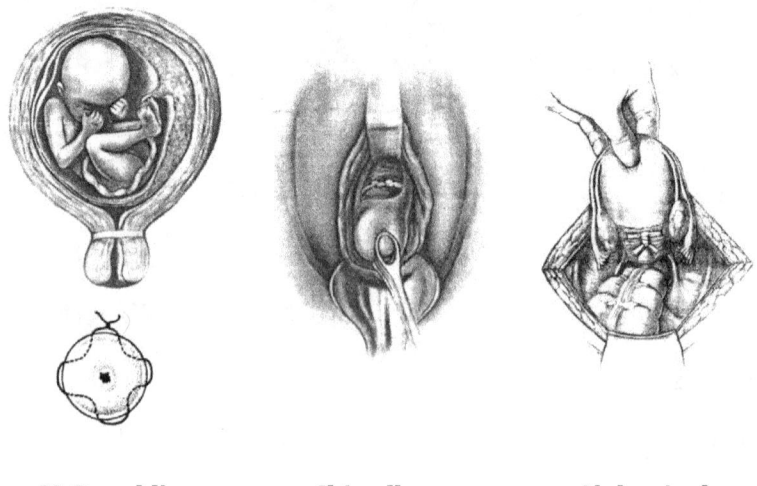

McDonald's   **Shirodkar**   **Abdominal**

ECTOPIC PREGNANCY

Definitions

- Pregnancy which develops outside the uterine cavity

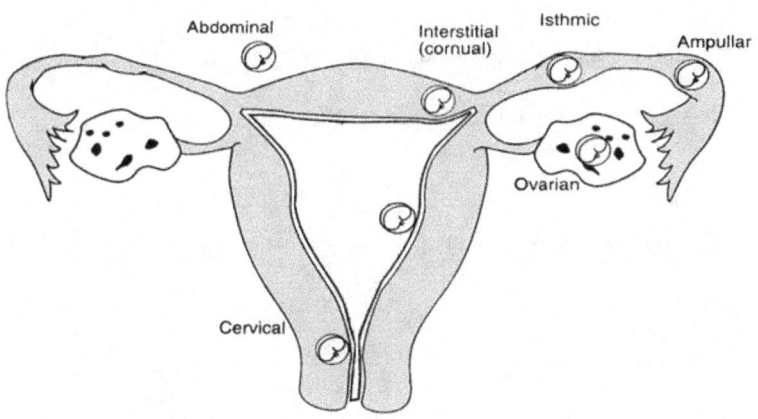

Types

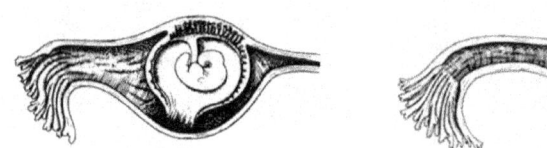

Non-ruptured   **Ruptured**

Causes

- Tubal surgery

- Pelvic inflammatory diseases

- Endometriosis

- Prior ectopic pregnancy

Diagnosis

- <u>Non-ruptured:</u>

• Unilateral pelvic pain in early amenorrhea

• Vaginal bleeding

• Unilateral tender mass and tender cervix on mobilization

• Endo-uterine darkish bleeding on speculum

- <u>Ruptured:</u>

• Abdominal pain of sudden onset in early amenorrhea

• Hypovolemic shock

• Abdominal rebound sign

• Douglas tenderness

Complications

- Severe anemia

- Hypovolemic shock

Investigations

- ß-HCG and doubling time

- Obstetric ultrasound

- Laparoscopy

Management

- Stabilize the patient hemodynamically

- <u>Surgical intervention:</u> (laparotomy / laparoscopy)

- <u>Medical treatment:</u> (Methotrexate)

• Hemodynamically stable

• Not ruptured

• Absence of embryo cardiac activity

• On ultrasound: Sac < 3 cm

• ß-HCG < 15,000 mIU / ml

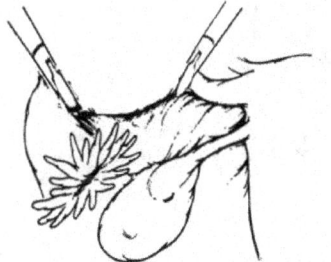 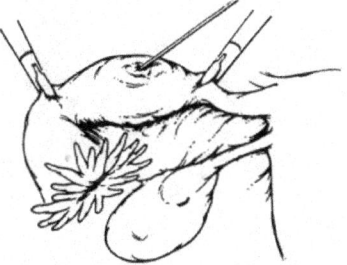

Salpingectomy   **Salpingotomy**

MOLAR PREGNANCY

Definition

- Trophoblastic disease characterised by abnormal proliferation of the trophoblastic cells with vesicular chorionic villi transformation

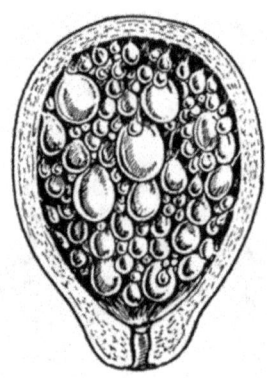

Types

- Complete mole

- Partial mole

Causes

- Chromosomal abnormality

Diagnosis

- Amenorrhea

- Vaginal bleeding and expulsion of vesicles

- Hyperemesis gravidarum

- The uterus is soft and large and ovaries are cystic

Complications

- Invasive mole

- Choriocarcinoma

- Hypertensive disorders of pregnancy

Investigations

- ß-HCG: higher than normal pregnancy

- Obstetric ultrasound: "Snow storm" appearance

Management

- Resuscitation if necessary

- Aspiration under ultrasound guidance

- Oxytocin after aspiration

- Post molar surveillance:

• Monitor levels of ß-HCG every week till 3 negative results, then every month for 2 years + combined OCPs (to prevent pregnancy)

• If ß-HCG is high, more likely invasive mole or choriocarcinoma which require chemotherapy

PLACENTA PREVIA

Definition

- The placenta is partially or completely implanted in the lower segment

of the uterus after viability

Types

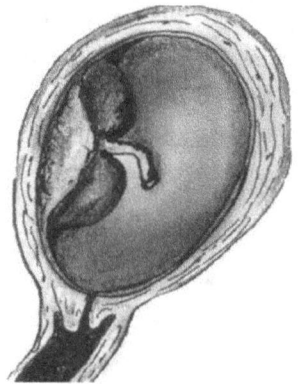

Low lying (lateralis)

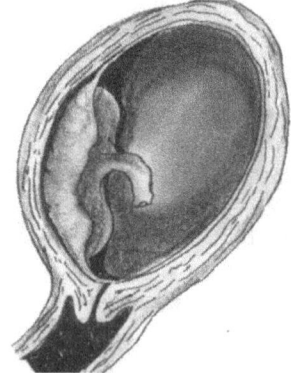

Marginalis

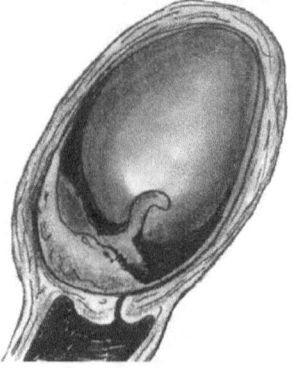

Incomplete centralis

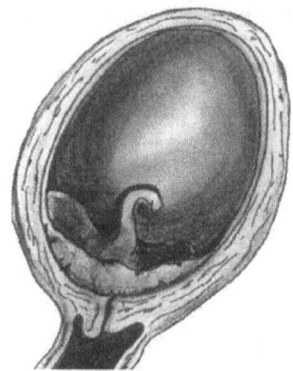

Complete centralis

Causes

- Advanced maternal age and high parity

- Deficient endometrium (uterine scar, CS ...)

- Large placental area (multiple pregnancies ...)

- Uterine malformations

- Prior placenta previa

Diagnosis

- Sudden onset of bright red fresh painless hemorrhage

- Unusual irritability and tenderness

- Often malpresentation of the fetus

- Endo-uterine cavity hemorrhage on speculum examination

Complications

- Anemia

- Hemorrhagic shock

- Malpresentations

- Prematurity

- Fetal distress

- IUFD

Investigations

- Complete blood count

- Obstetric ultrasound

Management

- <u>Expectant management:</u> (minimal hemorrhage, no uterine contractions)

• Bed rest

• Follow up

- <u>Active management:</u> (severe hemorrhage, uterine contractions)

• Placenta previa centralis: perfom CS.

• Placenta preavia marginalis: carefully perform amniotomy for vaginal delivery if the head is engaged.

PLACENTAL ABRUPTION

Definition

- Bleeding from the placental site due to premature separation of a normally situated placenta after viability

Types

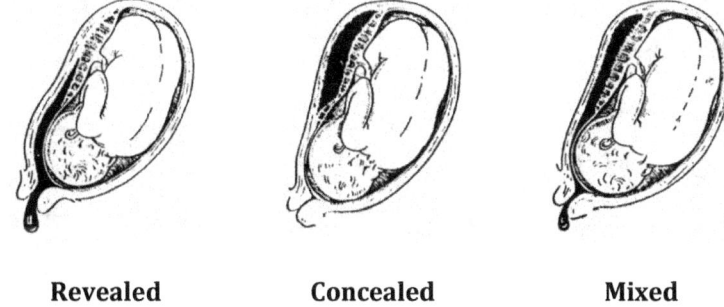

| Revealed | Concealed | Mixed |

Causes

- Severe pre-eclampsia

- Sudden rupture of membranes

- Short umbilical cord

- Trauma

- Dietary cause / smoking

Diagnosis

- Abdominal pain is moderate to severe but may be absent in small bleeds

- Vaginal bleeding: may pass dark blood or may be concealed

- The uterus is often very tender, painful and some times hard

Complications

- Hemorrhagic shock

- Coagulation disorders

- Renal failure

- Fetal distress

- IUFD

Investigations

- Coagulation profile

- Renal function tests

- Obstetric ultrasound: fetal well being, retroplacental hematoma

Management

- Maternal resuscitation:

• Shock

• DIC

- Obstetric management:

• If the fetus is alive: emergency CS

• If the fetus is dead: vaginal delivery is preferable (oxytocin infusion and

artificial rupture of membrane)

PRE-ECLAMPSIA

Definition

- Blood pressure of $\geq$ 140 / 90 mm Hg after 20 weeks of gestation plus proteinuria and / or edema

Causes

- Unknown

- Maternal age: < 20 and > 40 years

- Nulliparity

- Family history

- Pre-eclampsia in previous pregnancy

- Molar pregnancy

- Multiple gestation

- Chronic hypertension

- Diabetes mellitus

- Chronic renal disease

Diagnosis

- Blood pressure of $\geq$ 140 / 90 mm Hg

- Proteinuria ($\geq$ 300 mg / L)

- Generalised edema

- Headache, blurred vision, vomiting, epigastric pain

Complications

- <u>Maternal:</u>

• Eclampsia

• Abruption placenta

• Renal failure

• HELLP syndrome

• DIC

• Pulmonary edema

- <u>Fetal:</u>

• IUGR

• Prematurity

• IUFD

Investigations

- Complete blood count and coagulation profile

- Kidney function tests

- Liver function tests

- Obstetric ultrasound and Doppler

Management

- <u>Mild pre-eclampsia:</u>

• If preterm: close monitoring

• If at term: consider delivery

- <u>Severe pre-eclampsia:</u> (BP ≥ 160 / 110 mm Hg and / or proteinuria ≥ 5 g / 24 h)

• Anti-convulsion treatment:

Magnesium sulphate

Loading Dose: 6 g IV infusions

Maintenance dose: 4 g / 4 h IV infusions or IM

Monitor respiratory rate, urine output, and deep tendon reflexes

• Anti-hypertensive treatment:

Hydralazine IV

Labetalol if hypertension is refractory to hydralazine

• Obstetric management:

If preterm: give Dexamethasone and deliver by induction

If at term: deliver immediately preferably vaginal

ECLAMPSIA

Definition

- Onset of convulsion in a woman with pre-eclampsia that can not be attributed to other causes

Causes

- As Pre-eclampsia

Diagnosis

- Signs of severe pre-eclampsia

- Hypertension: > 160 / 110 mm Hg

- Tonic-clonic seizures

- Coma

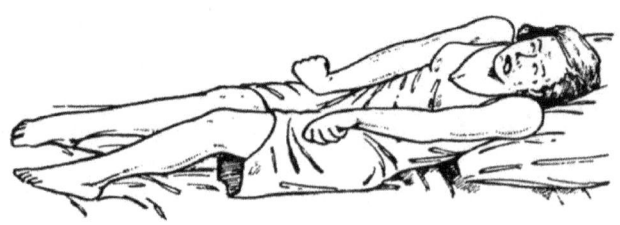

Complications

- Maternal:

• Renal Failure

• HELLP syndrome

• DIC

- Acute pulmonary oedema

- Heart failure

- Cerebral hemorrhage

- Retinal detachment

- <u>Fetal:</u>

- IUGR

- Prematurity

- IUFD

Investigations

- As Pre-eclampsia

Management

- Prevent aspiration and trauma during convulsions

- Give O_2 by face mask

- Insert 2 IV lines

- Fluids should be restricted to avoid pulmonary edema

- Insert a urinary catheter

- Anti-convulsion treatment: as severe pre-eclampsia

- Anti-hypertensive treatment: as severe pre-eclampsia

- Immediate delivery after stabilization should be considered

DIABETES MELLITUS

Definition

- Glucose intolerance caused by absolute or relative insulin deficiency

Causes

- Pre-existing diabetes: including type1, type 2

- A family history of gestational diabetes

- Obesity: BMI $\geq$ 30

- Age: > 40 years

- Previous pregnancy with diabetes and / or macrosomia

- Habitual abortion or IUFD

Diagnosis

- Excessive hunger

- Excessive thirst

- Excessive urination

- Recurrent vaginal infections (especially Candida infections)

- Tiredness

Complications

- Maternal:

• Abortion

• Pre-eclampsia

• Polyhydramnios

• Infection

• Preterm labor

• Diabetic keto-acidosis

• Hypoglycemia

• Deteriorating retinopathy, neuropathy

- Fetal:

• Macrosomia with traumatic delivery, shoulder dystocia

• Congenital malformations

• Sudden IUFD

• Respiratory distress syndrome

• Hypoglycemia at birth

• Hypocalcemia

• Polycythemia

• Jaundice

Investigations

- Screening 50 gm Oral Glucose Tolerance Test (OGTT): between 24-28

  weeks of pregnancy

- Diagnostic 100 gm OGTT: if abnormal 50 gm test

- Obstetric ultrasound and Doppler

- Retinal funduscopy

Management

- Carefully planned diet and exercise

- Oral antidiabetic drugs should be avoided during first trimester

- Daily insulin injections and monitoring glucose levels

- Induce labor or plan elective CS between 38-39 weeks of gestation

- Sliding scale is used to control the glucose level throughout labor

- Control glucose levels postpartum

CARDIAC DISEASE

Definition

- Cardiac disease may be associated with 0.5-1% of pregnancies

Causes

- Rheumatic heart valve diseases

- Congenital heart disease

- Coronary heart disease and cardiomyopathy

Diagnosis

- New York Heart Association (NYHA) grading:

• Class I: Organic heart disease without symptoms on ordinary activity

• Class II: Symptoms (dyspnea and chest pain) at ordinary activity

• Class III: Symptoms at less than ordinary activity

• Class IV: Dyspnea at rest

Complications

- Abortion

- IUGR

- Preterm labor

Investigations

- ECG

- Echocardiography

Management

- Semi-sitting position

- Adequate oxygenation

- Proper pain relief

- Straining is prohibited

- Antibiotic cover to guard against SBE

- Digitalis in cases at high risk for heart failure

- Shorten the second stage by low-forceps when necessary

- Ergometrine is given only if postpartum hemorrhage occurs

- CS is done when obstetrically indicated

ASYMPTOMATIC BACTERIURIA

Definition

- Bacterial count > 100,000 / ml in 2 midstream freshly voided urine samples

Causes

- Most commonly: Gram-negative bacteria (E.coli …)

- Less commonly: Gram-positive cocci (Staphylococci …)

- Gravidity: hormonal and urine stasis

Diagnosis

- Often asymptomatic

Complications

- Acute pyelonephritis

- Preterm labor

Investigations

- Urine analysis / culture and sesetivity

- Renal function tests

Management

- Increase water intake

- Antibiotics based on culture and sensitivity

ACUTE PYELONEPHRITIS

Definition

- Acute pyelonephritis during pregnancy, most often, is a complication of

  non-treated asymptomatic bacteriuria

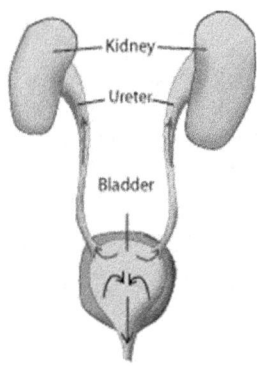

Causes

- As asymptomatic bacteriuria

Diagnosis

- Headache, fever, chills, nausea and / or vomiting

- Flank pain and dysuria

Complications

- Chronic renal failure

- Recurrence

- Preterm labor

- IUFD

Investigations

- Urine analysis

- Urine culture

- Renal function tests

Management

- Rest

- Increase water intake

- Analgesics

- Antipyretics

- Antibiotics based on culture and sensitivity

HYPEREMESIS GRAVIDARUM

Definition

- Severe nausea and vomiting in early pregnancy requiring hospital admission and rehydration

Causes

- Hormonal: high levels of β-HCG like in multiple pregnancy and hydatiforme mole.

- Emotional: psychological and social factors

- Endocrine disorders: adrenocortical insufficiency

Diagnosis

- Nausea and vomiting typically in early pregnancy

- Dehydration

- Weight loss

- Altered general status (tachycardia, hypotension)

Complications

- Metabolic disorders (hyponatraemia, hypokalaemia, hypochloremic alkalosis, ketonuria) that may lead to coma

- Jaundice

- Neurological disorders (Wernicke's encephalopathy)

- Retinal hemorrhage

Investigations

- Blood for urea, electrolytes and serum creatinine

- Kidney function tests

- Liver function tests

- Obstetric ultrasound

Management

- Isolation

- Reassure the mother

- Monitor diuresis

- Monitor electrolytes

- NPO for 48 hours

- Intravenous rehydration: alternate Ringers lactate with normal saline

- Antiemetics

- Corticosteroids

- Vitamin B1 and B6

- Termination of pregnancy in severe cases with failed treatment

ANEAMIA

Definition

Hemoglobin levels that fall < 11 g / dl

Causes

- Low intake of iron and folic acid

- Repeated pregnancies

- Repeated blood loss associated with pregnancy

- Sickle cell anemia

Diagnosis

- Dizziness, faintness, headache

- Dyspnea, palpitations

- Tiredness, weakness

- Pale color of skin and mucous membranes

Complications

- Abortion

- IUGR

- Premature labor

- IUFD

- PPH

- Infections

Investigations

- Complete blood count

- Blood cross-match

- Red cell morphology

- Red blood cell electrophoresis

- Iron studies

Management

- Determine the cause of anemia and treat accordingly

- Iron rich diet

- Hb > 7 gm / dl: start iron and vitamin supplements

- Hb < 7gm / dl: blood transfusion

THROMBOEMBOLISM

Definitions

- Deep Vein Thrombosis (DVT): formation of blood clots within the deep veins, most commonly in the lower extremities or pelvis

- Pulmonary Embolus (PE): thrombosis or showers of emboli in the pulmonary vessels

Pregnancy-associated Causes

- Changes in local clotting factors

- Mechanical impedance of venous return

- Vessel damage during pregnancy

Risk Factors

- Advanced maternal age

- Increased parity

- Multiple pregnancy

- Surgery: CS, episiotomy, lacerations ...

- Prolonged immobility

- Dehydration

- Prior DVT or PE

- Lupus anticoagulant.

- Pre-eclampsia

Diagnosis

- Pain or tenderness, fever

- Asymmetric limb swelling, > 2 cm larger than opposite side

- Warmth or erythema of skin over area of thrombosis

- Homan's sign: calf pain with dorsiflexion of the foot

- With PE: tachycardia, dyspnea and chest pain

- Death with massive PE

Complications

- Septic pelvic thrombophlebitis

- Death

- Recurrent PE

- Pulmonary hypertention

Investigations

- Complete blood count

- Coagulation profile: PTT, PT / INR

- Renal function tests

- Liver function tests

- Obstetric ultrasound, Doppler

- CT scan

- Chest X-ray

- Angiography

Management

- Bed rest

- Graduated elastic compression stocking should be applied

- Inferior vena cava filter can be used to avoid PE

- Enoxaparin: 1 mg / kg SC every 12 hours for the acute phase

- Enoxaparin can be substituted with heparin

- Warfarin: 5-7.5 mg loading dose and then the maintainence dose will depend on INR results for 6 weeks

- Acetylsalicylic acid (aspirin): 75-100 mg daily to be continued up to 6 weeks postpartum

- Avoid hormonal contraception; risk increases with estrogen containing contraceptions

- For the next pregnancy: anticoagulation therapy throught pregnancy

THYROTOXICOSIS

Diagnosis

- Clinical manifestations

Complications

- Fetal hyper or hypothyroidism

- Fetal goiter, face or brow presentation

Investigations

- Thyroid functions

Management

- Propylthiouracil and β-blockers

- Thyroidectomy if indicated

TOXOPLASMOSIS

Causes

- An infection caused by a single cell parasite called "Toxoplasma gondii", found in the domestic cats

- Eating raw or undercooked meat or ingesting soil contaminated with Toxoplasma gondii oocysts, which are excreted in the faeces of infected cats

Diagnosis

- Asymptomatic or flu-like symptoms

- Fever

- Malaise

- Lymphadenopathy

- Neurological involvement in immunocompromized

Complications

- Congenital abnormalities (chorioretinitis, blindness, hydrocephalus ...)

- IUGR

- IUFD

Investigations

- Toxoplasmosis serology (IgG, IgM in 1st trimester if possible)

- Ultrasound to detect abnormalities

Management

- Advice the patient not to eat raw / uncooked food

- Attention to domestic cats

- Spiramycin (Rovamycin)

- Pyrimethamine (not in the first trimester as it is folic acid antagonist)

  and Sulfadiazine

RUBELLA

Causes

- Rubella virus (RNA)

- Droplet infection by naso-pharengeal secretions

Diagnosis

- Asymptomatic or flu-like symptoms

- Fever

- Malaise

- Lymphadenopathy

Complications

- Congenital rubella syndrome (cataract, deafness, PDA ...)

- IUGR

- IUFD

Investigations

- IgG, IgM in 1st trimester if possible

- Ultrasound to detect abnormalities

Management

- Rubella vaccine (live attenuated): before pregnancy

- If exposure in the first trimester: termination of pregnancy

CYTOMEGALOVIRUS

Causes

- Cytomegalovirus (CMV)

- Sexual or respiratory contact with infected secretions

Diagnosis

- Asymptomatic or flu-like symptoms

- Fever

- Malaise

- Lymphadenopathy

Complications

- Congenital abnormalities (cataract, deafness, PDA ...)

- IUGR

- IUFD

Investigations

- Culture from secretions

- Serology

- Ultrasound to detect abnormalities

Management

- If exposure in the first trimester: termination of pregnancy

HERPES SIMPLEX VIRUS

Causes

- Genital herpes is caused by the herpes simplex virus either type 1 or 2 (HSV-1 or HSV-2)

- During primary infection of HSV the mother can infect the fetus during delivery

Diagnosis

- Painful lesions on labia, clitoris, perinium, vagina and cervix

- Vesicles, shallow ulcers

- Inguinal lymph nodes

Complications

- Viral pneumonia for the mother

- Mother-to-child transmission

- Abortion

- Preterm labor

- CNS defect

- Neonatal death

Investigations

- HSV genital culture

- Serology for HSV

Management

- Analgesics

- Acyclovir

- Gentian violet

- Advise the pregnant mother that CS is preferable in cases of primary genital infections

- If spontaneous rupture of the membranes occurs, CS should be performed as soon as possible, particularly within 4 hours

SYPHILLIS

Causes

- It is a sexual transmitted infection caused by spirochaetes "Treponema pallidum" which can infect the fetus at any point in the gestation

Diagnosis

- Primary stage: (incubation usually 3 weeks)

• Chancre on the genital area

• Regional lymphadenopathy

- Secondary stage: (7-10 weeks after exposure)

• Skin manifestations: hands, chest, labia, clitoris, lips ...

• Fever, headache, generalized lymphadenopathy

- Tertiary stage: (10-20 years after primary infection)

• Gumma lesions

• Cardiovascular disease: aortic aneurysm and aortic insufficiency

• Neurological involvement, general paresis, tabes dorsalis

Complications

- Abortion

- Prematurity

- IUFD

- Congenital syphilis: muco-cutaneous lesions, bone and visceral lesions

Investigations

- <u>Microscopy:</u> by dark field examination

- <u>Serology:</u>

• Nonspecific treponemal tests: VDRL or RPR

• Specific treponemal tests: TPHA or FTA-Ab

Management

- Benzathine penicillin: 2.4 million IU IM weekly for three consecutive weeks

- Allergic to penicillin must be desensitized and treated

- Erythromycin: 500 mg / 6 h for 14 days, but may not prevent congenital syphilis

HEPATITIS B VIRUS

Causes

- Hepatitis B is a viral disease of liver transmitted by:

• Blood

• Sexual intercource

• Vertical transmission

Diagnosis

- Incubation period: 6 weeks - 6 months

- Most of the time asymptomatic

- Symptoms: (in 0.5% cases)

• Jaundice, tiredness, dark urine

• Liver cirrhosis and failure

Complications

- Liver cirrhosis and failure

- Hepatocellurar carcinoma

- Mother to child transmission

- Abortion

- IUGR

- prematurity

- IUFD

Investigations

- HBs Ag

- HBeAg (e antigen identifies a high infective status)

- Anti-HBe (anti-HBe or HBeAb)

- HBV viral load (HBV DNA)

- Liver function test

Management

- Exposed patients: are given Hepatitis B vaccine and Hepatitis B immunoglobulin during pregnancy

- Intrapartum management:

• There is no evidence that CS reduces the risk of perinatal transmission

• Avoid procedures that may inoculate the baby

- Care of the newborn:

• Hepatitis B vaccine and Hepatitis B immunoglobulin

• Breast-feeding is not contraindicated

HEPATITIS C VIRUS

Causes

- Hepatitis C is a viral disease of liver transmitted by:

• Blood

• Sexual intercource

• Vertical transmission

Diagnosis

- Incubation period: 6-10 weeks

- The acute hepatitis may not be diagnosed as symptoms are mild

- Headache, malaise, lethargy

- Right upper quadrant pain

- Jaundice

- Liver cirrhosis and failure

Complications

- Liver cirrhosis and failure

- Hepatocellurar carcinoma

Investigations

- Ac-anti HcVirus

- Hepatitis C RNA PCR

- Liver function tests

Management

- <u>Routine screening:</u> for hepatitis C antibodies

- <u>Intrapartum management:</u>

• There is no evidence that CS reduces the risk of perinatal transmission

• Avoid procedures that may inoculate the baby

- <u>Breast-feeding:</u> is not contraindicated

HUMAN IMMUNODEFICIENCY VIRUS

Causes

- Transmission of human immunodeficiency virus (HIV) from the infected mother to child may occur during pregnancy, labor, and breastfeeding especially with:

• High Viral load

• Low CD 4 cell count

• Prolonged labor

Investigations

- Serologic test for HIV

- CD4 count, viral load

Management

- Prevention

- Pregnant HIV positive women are eligible to ART e.g. Azidothymidine (AZT) from 14 weeks of gestation for life

OLIGOHYDRAMNIOS

Definition

- Amniotic fluid volume < 5th percentile for gestational age or < 500 ml

- By ultrasound: largest amniotic fluid pocket < 1 cm or AFI < 5

Causes

- Fetal congenital anomalies: renal anomalies are the most common

- Placental insufficiency

- Undiagnosed PROM

Diagnosis

- History of leaking amniotic fluid in PROM

- The patient does not feal progressive abdominal enlargement

- Decreased fundal level in relation to gestational age

Complications

- Abortion

- IUGR

- Preterm labor

- Pulmonary hypoplasia

- Contracture limb deformities

- Amniotic band formation

- Umbilical cord compression causing fetal hypoxia

Investigations

- Obstetric ultrasound:

• Largest amniotic fluid pocket < 1 cm

• AFI < 5

Management

- Pregnancy termination: concidered in patients with placental insufficiency or lethal fetal congenital anomalies e.g. renal agenesis

- Amnio-infusion: repeated injection of saline into the uterus via amniocentesis or trancervical infusion

POLYHYDRAMNIOS

Definition

- Amniotic fluid volume > 95th percentile for gestational age or > 2000 ml

- By ultrasound: largest amniotic fluid pocket > 8 cm or AFI > 25

Causes

- Fetal:

• Twins especially uniovular with twin to twin transfusion syndrome

• Fetal anomalies as anencephaly and esophageal

• Placental chorioangioma

• Large placenta

- Maternal:

• Pre-eclampsia: due to placental edema

• Diabetes mellitus: due to increased osmolarity of the amniotic fluid

• Severe generalized edema: cardiac, renal or nutritional.

Diagnosis

- Progressive abdominal enlargement

- Pressure symptoms

- Fundal level is higher than expected for the period of amenorrhea

- Fetal parts are difficult to feel

- Fluid thrill may be elicited

Complications

- Pressure symptoms

- Malpresentations

- Abortion

- Accidental haemorrhage if ROM occurs suddenly

- Pre-eclampsia

- Preterm labor

- Prolonged labor

- PROM

- Cord presentation and prolapse

- Postpartum haemorrhage

- Postpartum infection

Investigations

- Obstetric ultrasound:

• Largest amniotic fluid pocket > 8 cm

• AFI > 25

• Twins

• Fetal anomalies

Management

- Establishing the cause if present

- Rest

- Indomethacin: decreases fetal urine production

- Amniocentesis: Removing up to 1.5 to 2 litres of amniotic fluid, via inserting a needle trans-abdominally under ultrasound guidance

- Termination of pregnancy: if > 37 weeks

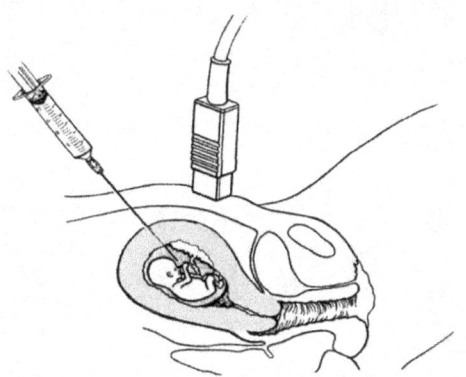

Amniocentesis

INTRAUTERINE GROWTH RESTRICTION

Definition

- Intrauterine growth restriction (IUGR) or small for gestational age (SGA) is a fetal weight that is below the 10th percentile for gestational age as determined by ultrasound

Types

- Symetrical

- Asymetrical

Causes

- Maternal factors:

• Preeclampsia

• Chronic hypertension

• Diabetes in pregnancy

• Cardiac disorders

• Renal disease

• Anemia

• Coagulopathies (thrombophilias).

• Poor nutrition

• Respiratory disease (severe asthma …)

• Anti-phospholipid syndrome

- Fetal factors:

• Multiple pregnancy

• Fetal infection

• Chromosomal defects

• Malformations

- Placental factors:

• Placental cysts

• Chorioangioma

• Placenta previa

• Thrombosis, infarction

• Decreased uteroplacental blood flow

- Uterine factors:

• Uterine abnormalities (especially uterine septum)

• Fibromyoma (large submucosal fibroids)

Diagnosis

- Symptoms of the cause: preeclampsia, diabetes ...

- Small fundal height for gestational age

Complications

- Fetal distress

- IUFD

- Meconium stained liquor

Investigations

- Ultrasound findings: < 10th percentile estimated fetal weight

- Biophysical profile

- Umbilical artery Doppler

- CTG

Management

- Proper pregnancy dating

- Treatment of the cause

- <u>If end diastolic flow is present:</u> delay delivery after 37 weeks

- <u>If end diastolic flow is absent:</u>

• Baby > 34 weeks: consider delivery

• Baby < 34 weeks: patient should be admitted and monitored by CTG, receiving corticosteroids and consider delivery after 48 hours by CS

- If vaginal delivery, continous CTG is a mandatory

- Suctioning pharynx as soon as possible after delivery to avoid meconium aspiration

POST-TERM PREGNANCY

Definition

- Pregnancy lasting beyond 42 weeks from the first day of the LMP

Causes

- Error in dating

- Primigravida

- Anencephaly

Complications

- Fetal distress / meconium stained liquor

- Dysmaturity syndrome

- Fetal macrosomia

Investigations

- Obstetric ultrasound

- Umbilical artery Doppler

Management

- Proper pregnancy dating

- Induction of labor: if no contraindication

- CS: if failure of induction or fetal distress

PRETERM LABOR

Definition

- Preterm labor is occurance of uterine contractions before 37 weeks of gestation

Causes

- History of previous preterm birth

- Adolescent age and advanced maternal age

- Maternal infections: acute pyelonephritis, genital tract infection, other systemic infections ...

- Increased uterine size: twins, polyhydramnios ...

- Maternal trauma

- Uterine abnormalities: malformations, myomas ...

- Other pregnancy complications: cervical incompetence, abruption placentae ...

- Social, economic and stress factors

Diagnosis

- Pelvic and back pain

- Uterine contractions

- Increased vaginal discharge / leaking of amniotic fluid

- Muco-bloody discharge

Investigations

- Urine analysis

- Vaginal swab for analysis

- Materanl and fetal screening for infections

- Obstetric ultrasound

Complications

- Prematurity

- Neonatal respiratory distress syndrome

- Neonatal mortality and morbidity

Management

- Cervix dilatation < 4 cm:

• Tocolysis:

  B2 agonists (Ritodrine HCL) or

  Calcium channel blockers (Nifedipine)

• Monitor maternal heart rate (it should not go up 120 / min)

• Dexamethasone 6 mg IM 4 doses 12 hourly for lung maturity

• Delivery should be delayed for 24 to 48 hours

- Cervix dilatation ≥ 4 cm:

• Tocolysis: B2 agonists or Nifedipine for 24 hours

• Dexamethasone: 12 mg IM 2 doses 12 hourly

• This will assist transfer to a center with good neonatology facilities

- <u>During labor:</u>

• Continuous electronic monitoring of the fetus during labor is mandatory because preterm infants tolerate hypoxia more poorly than term infants

• Avoid prolongation of the 2nd stage of labor

• Episiotomy: to prevent head compression and ICH

• CS is indicated in preterm breech, and the extremely LBW fetus

• Neonates should be transferred to neonatology unit

• Next pregnancy is at high risk for preterm labor and should be closely monitored

PREMATURE RUPTURE OF MEMBRANES

Definitions

- Premature rupture of membranes (PROM): rupture of fetal membranes prior to onset of labor

- Preterm premature rupture of membranes (PPROM): rupture of fetal membranes prior to onset of labor prior to 37 weeks

Causes

- Maternal infections (pyelonephritis, genital tract infection ...).

- Cervical incompetence

- Increased uterine size: twins, polyhydramnios ...

Diagnosis

- Sudden gush of fluid from the vagina followed by intermittent trickle

- Sterile speculum examination to confirm leaking of amniotic fluid

- Nitrazine test to detect the alkaline pH of amniotic fluid in the vagina

Investigations

- Complete blood count

- Urine analysis

- Vaginal swab for analysis

- Materanl and fetal screening for infections

- Obstetric ultrasound

Complications

- Infection: chorioamnionitis, neonatal sepsis, maternal septicemia ...

- Prematurity

- Neonatal respiratory distress syndrome

- Neonatal mortality and morbidity

Management

- <u>Termination of pregnancy:</u> (irrespective of gestational age)

• Clinical and laboratory evidence of chorioamnionitis

• Fetal condition is not reassuring

- <u>PROM (> 37 weeks):</u>

• Termination of pregnancy under cover of suitable antibiotics and close fetal monitoring

• Spontaneous labor will start within 24-48 hours in 80-90% of cases

- <u>PPROM (< 37 weeks):</u>

• Prophylactic antibiotics given to guard against infection

• Corticosteroids may be given in cases < 34 weeks

CHORIOAMNIONITIS

Definition

- Bacterial infection of amniotic fluid and fetal membranes

- It typically complicates PROM and results from bacterial ascending into the uterus from the vagina

Causes

- PROM

- Genital tract infections

- Urinary tract Infection

Diagnosis

- Fever

- Tachycardia (maternal and fetal)

- Uterine tenderness

- Foul-smelling discharge

Complications

- Fetal distress

- IUFD

- Neonatal Infection

- Endometritis

- Septicemia, septic shock

Investigations

- Complete blood count

- CRP

- Urine analysis

- Vaginal swab

- Cervical cultures

- Fluid leakage culture

- Obstetric ultrasound

Management

- Antibiotics: Ampicillin and Metronidazole

- Vaginal delivery is preferred

RHESUS ISOIMMUNIZATION

Definition

- Rhesus isoimmunization is the condition where incompatibility exists between the fetal and maternal rhesus group such that an immune response occurs

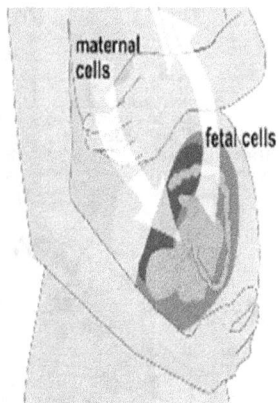

Causes

- Delivery

- Abortion

- Ectopic pregnancy

- Hydatiforme mole

- Abruption placenta

- Invasive procedures

- Other causes of bleeding during pregnancy

Complications

- Recurrent abortion

- Fetal anemia

- Hydrops fetalis (defined as an abnormal collection of fluid in two or more fetal body compartments, including ascites, pleural effusions, pericardial effusions, and skin edema)

- Intrauterine fetal death

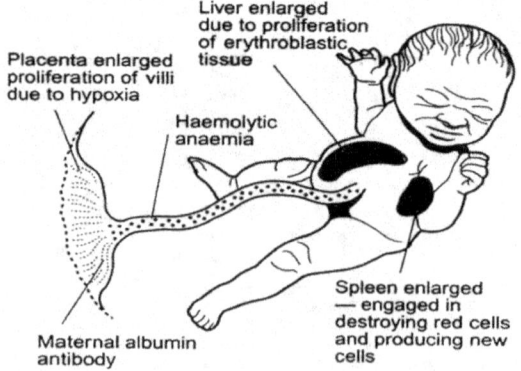

Liver enlarged due to proliferation of erythroblastic tissue

Placenta enlarged proliferation of villi due to hypoxia

Haemolytic anaemia

Spleen enlarged — engaged in destroying red cells and producing new cells

Maternal albumin antibody

Investigations

- <u>Antibody titers:</u> serial measurements of circulating antibody titers should be performed every 2-4 weeks

- <u>Invasive testing:</u> if antibody titers continue to rise in the presence of an Rh (D)-positive fetus, invasive testing may be required

• Amniocentesis

• Fetal blood sampling for fetal hemoglobin

Management

- Rhesus (anti-D) prophylaxis:

• 300 IU Anti-rhesus Immunoglobulin

• At 28-32 weeks' gestation

• Within 72 hours after delivery if the baby is Rh (D)-positive

- Monitoring the pregnancy: blood group (ABO and Rh) and antibody status testing at booking

- Blood transfusion: in case of fetal anemia unless fetal hydrops is already present

- Timing of delivery: at $\geq$ 34 weeks of gestation in case of complications

FETAL ANOMALIES

Causes

- Congenital anomalies:

• Structural anomalies: e.g. neural tube defects (NTDs)

• Biochemical anomalies: e.g. phenylketonuria

- Chromosomal anomalies: e.g. Down syndrome (trisomy 21)

Diagnosis

- Maternal age more than 35 years

- Exposure to certain infections

- Administration of teratogenic drugs or chemicals

- Exposure to irradiation especially during early pregnancy

- One or both parents with a defined chromosomal anomal

- Past history of previous affected fetus

- Obstetric history of successive spontaneous abortions

Investigations

- Maternal serum screening:

• Alpha fetoprotein (AFP): rises in neural tube defects (NTDs) and turner syndrome, and decreases in trisomy 21 (Down syndrome)

• Triple marker test: risk of Down syndrome is high when decreased MSAFP and uE3 levels, and increased levels of HCG

- Ultrasound screening:

• Anencephaly can be excluded by the end of first trimester.

• Other neural tube defects (NTDs), most of the skeletal, cardiac, renal and GIT anomalies can be efficiently diagnosed in the second trimester.

• Nuchal translucency (NT)

- Amniocentesis

- Chorionic villous sampling (CVS)

- Cordocentesis

- Fetoscopy

- Magnetic resonance imaging (MRI)

- Preimplantation genetic diagnosis (PGD)

Management

- In utero fetal therapy in selected cases (if possible)

- Counseling the parents about termination of pregnancy (only if anomaly is lethal) with identification of any possible maternal hazards

- Preparation for postnatal treatment of the newborn

FETAL ASPHYXIA

Definition

- Fetal asphyxia is a state of inadequate oxygenation and inadequate elimination of CO_2, which may result in metabolic acidemia (umbilical arterial blood pH < 7.2)

Causes

- Maternal factors:

• Maternal age: > 40 or < 16 years

• Pregnancy induced hypertension

• Diabetes

• Renal disease

• Severe anemia

• Infections

• Use of narcotics

- Fetal factors:

• Multiple pregnancy

• Oligohydramnios and polyhydramnios

• IUGR

• Post-term

• Macrosomia

• Prematurity

• Isoimmunisation and hydrops fetalis

• Intrauterine infections

• Congenital malformation

- Pregnancy and labor factors:

• Malpresentations and malposition

• Antepartum hemorrhage

• Post-term pregnancy

• Prolonged PROM

• Fetal distress

• Meconium-stained liquor

• General anesthesia

• Instrumental delivery

• Emergency CS

Diagnosis

- Daily fetal movement count (DFMC)

- Non stress test (NST)

- Contraction stress test (CST)

- Obstetric ultrasound

- Biophysical profile (BPP)

- Doppler ultrasound

- CTG: tachycardia, bradycardia, late deceleration, variable deceleration

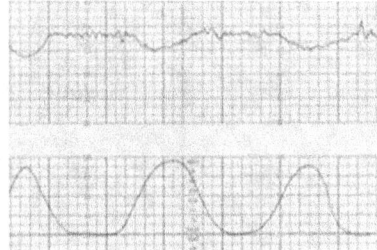 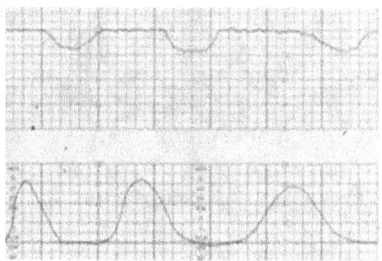

Early Deceleration   **Late Deceleration**

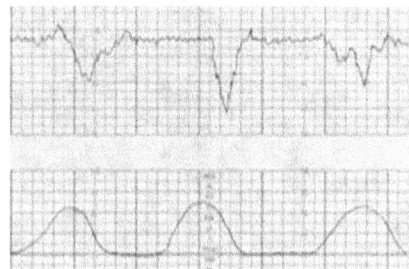

Variable Deceleration

- Fetal scalp pH (< 7.2)

- Mucous, blood or meconium in airway

- No breathing seen or felt

- No pulse felt at umbilical cord or no heart beat heard with sthetoscope

- APGAR < 7 at the 1st minute of life

Complications

- Cerebral palsy

- Neonatal death

Management

- <u>Proper antenatal care:</u>

• Treat the probable cause of intrauterine asphyxia if possible

• Fetal Surveillance

- <u>Proper intranatal care:</u>

• Careful observation of CTG.

• Avoid operative trauma.

• Episiotomy especially for breech and premature infants

• Aspiration of mucus and meconium from fetal larynx before breathing

- <u>Clearing air passages:</u>

• Holding the infant from the feet

• Aspirating mucus from mouth and upper pharynx by a rubber catheter

- <u>Warming the infant:</u>

• To decrease oxygen requirements

• To avoid attacks of apnea

- <u>Oxygen therapy:</u>

• Small mask or stream in front of the mouth and nose

• Endotracheal tube if indicated

- <u>Artificial respiration:</u>

• Endotracheal tube with intermittent positive pressure insufflation

• Mouth to mouth breathing until endotracheal tube is available

- <u>Cardiopulmonary resuscitation:</u>

• Cardiac resuscitation together with endotracheal entubation (or mouth to mouth breathing) if no audible heart beats or heart rate < 100

• Thumbs are put at the junction of lower and middle 1/3 of sternum to compress the chest gently 100 times / minute

- <u>Pharmaceutical management:</u>

• Adrenaline: 0.01-0.03 mg / kg IV, IM, ET

• Naloxone: 0.1 mg / kg IV, IM, SC, ET if narcotic analgesia was used during labor

• Normal Saline: 10 cc / kg IV over 5-10 minutes

• Dextrose: 10% 2 ml / kg

• Treat the underlying cause after stabilization

• Refer the infant to neonatology unit

MANAGEMENT OF HIGH RISK PREGNANCY

Definittion

- High risk pregnancy is a pregnancy complicated by a disease or a disorder that may affect the health or endanger the life of the mother or the fetus

Identification

- History:

• Age: whether young (< 18) or elderly (> 35) primigravida

• Parity: whether nullipara or grand multipara

• Previous obstetric difficulties, fetal loss or abnormalities

• Medical disorders as: diabetes, cardiac or renal disease

- General examination:

• Extreme obesity and short stature

• Hypertension

• Severe anemia, cardiac or renal disease

• Poor weight gain during pregnancy

- Obstetric examination:

• Malpresentations

• Multiple pregnancy

• Fetopelvic disproportion

• Antepartum hemorrhage

• Preeclampsia

- Investigations:

• Severe anemia, thrombocytopaenia, hyperglycaemia

• Rh negative blood typing

• Glycosuria and albuminuria

- Screening for infections:

• TORCH; toxoplasmosis, rubella, cytomegalovirus, herpes simplex

• Hepatitis B, C and HIV

- Screening for fetal anomalies:

• Congenital anomalies: NTDs, skeletal deformities, cardiac and renal anomalies, etc… (by ultrasound for fetal anatomy survey)

• Chromosomal anomalies: Down's syndrome (by 1st trimester maternal serum screening, ultrasound, CVS, 2nd trimester amniocentesis)

Management

- Preconception counseling: the obstetrician discusses and explains the following items

• The high risk factor(s) and its possible effects on the mother, fetus, and the newborn

• The importance of proper monitoring during pregnancy and labor

• The possibility of early intervention and the sequelae of preterm labor

- The need for antenatal care in a well equipped antenatal clinic

- The need to deliver in a well equipped hospital, with warning against home delivery

- Antenatal care:

- Once identified during preconception visit, first antenatal visit or return visits, the mother should be transferred for antenatal care and delivery in a specialized center ready for such high risk cases.

- Fetal surveillance:

- Correlation between fetal growth and gestational age (clinically and ultrasonography)

- Daily fetal movement count (DFMC)

- Non stress test (NST)

- Contraction stress test (CST)

- Biophysical profile (BPP) score

- Doppler ultrasound

- Delivery of high risk patients:

- Attention to the risks that may develop during labor

- The place of delivery should be fully equipped for maternal and fetal resuscitation (maternal and neonatal ICU)

- Efficient well-trained personnel, specialists and consultants should be available 24 hours a day

- Monitoring of fetal well being during labor, maternal condition and progress of labor (partogram) is essential

- Postnatal care:

- The mother is still at risk for complications during the immediate and late postpartum period

- The new born must be assessed and managed by a neonatologist

MATERNAL MORTALITY

Definitions

- Maternal mortality: maternal deaths due to obstetric causes (during pregnancy, delivery, or puerperium

- Maternal mortality rate (MMR): number of maternal deaths due to obstetric causes per 100,000 deliveries per year

Causes

- Antepartum haemorrhage

- Pregnancy induced hypertension

- Medical problems as heart disease with pregnancy

- Pulmonary embolism and DIC

- Postpartum hemorrhage

- Rupture of the uterus

- Infection: postpartum and postabortive

- Complications of anaesthesia

- Complications of CS

FETAL / NEONATAL MORTALITY

Definitions

- Intrauterine fetal death (IUFD): fetal death during pregnancy

- Intrapartum fetal death: fetal death during delivery

- Neonatal death: infant death in the first 4 weeks after delivery

- Perinatal mortality: includes intrauterine and intrapartum fetal deaths and neonatal death during the first week after delivery

Causes

- Intrauterine fetal death:

• Hypertensive disorders of pregnancy

• Diabetes with pregnancy

• Placental insufficiency

• True knots of the cord

• Rh incompatibility

• Congenital fetal anomalies

• Idiopathic (unexplained)

- Intrapartum fetal death:

• Asphyxia

• Birth trauma

• Intracranial hemorrhage

- <u>Neonatal death:</u>

• Prematurity

• Congenital fetal anomalies

• Neonatal asphyxia

• Birth injuries

• Hemolytic and hemorrhagic diseases of the newly born

• Respiratory distress syndrome

• Neonatal infection

REFERENCES

- 5-Minute Obstetrics and Gynecology Consult. Late pregnancy bleeding. 2009.

- Abalos E, Duley L, Steyn D. Antihypertensive drug therapy for mild to moderate hypertension during pregnancy. Cochrane Database Syst Rev 2014; 2: CD002252.

- Abalos E, Chamillard M, Diaz V, et al. Antenatal care for healthy pregnant women: a mapping of interventions from existing guidelines to inform the development of new WHO guidance on antenatal care. BJOG. 2016; 123: 519.

- ACOG Practice Bulletin no. 80. Premature rupture of membranes. Clinical management guidelines for obstetrician-gynecologists. Obstet Gynecol. 2007; 109: 1007-19.

- ACOG Practice Bulletin no. 106: Intrapartum fetal heart rate monitoring: nomenclature, interpretation, and general management principles. Obstet Gynecol 2009; 114: 192.

- ACOG Practice Bulletin no. 127: Management of preterm labor. Obstet Gynecol 2012; 119: 1308.

- ACOG Practice Bulletin no. 134: Fetal growth restriction. Obstet Gynecol 2013; 121: 1122.

- ACOG Practice Bulletin no. 175: Ultrasound in Pregnancy. Clinical management guidelines for obstetrician-gynecologists. Obstet Gynecol. 2016; 128: e241.

- Alfirevic Z, Devane D, Gyte G. Continuous cardiotocography (CTG) as a form of electronic fetal monitoring (EFM) for fetal assessment during labour. Cochrane Database Syst Rev. 2006; 3: CD006066.

- Alfirevic Z, Stampalija T, Gyte G. Fetal and umbilical Doppler ultrasound in high-risk pregnancies. Cochrane Database Syst Rev 2013; 11: CD007529.

- Attilakos G, Overton T. Antenatal Care, in Dewhurst's Textbook of Obstetrics and Gynaecology. 8th ed. Oxford, UK: Wiley-Blackwell; 2012.

- Baschat A. Fetal growth restriction - from observation to intervention. J Perinat Med. 2010; 38: 239.

- Beckmann C, Ling F, Barzansky B. Obstetrics and Gynecology. 4th ed. Philadelphia, Pa: Lippincott Williams & Wilkins; 2001.

- Centre for Disease Control and Prevention. Sexual ly transmitted disease treatment guidelines. 2006.

- Chauhan S, Taylor M, Shields D, et al. Intrauterine growth restriction and oligohydramnios among high-risk patients. Am J Perinatol. 2007; 24: 215.

- Creasy R, Resnik R, Iams J. Maternal-Fetal Medicine. In: Principles and Practice. 5th ed. Philadelphia, Pa: WB Saunders; 2004.

- Cunningham F, Leveno K, Bloom J, et al. Williams Obstetrics. 23rd ed. New York: McGraw-Hill; 2010.

- Figueras F, Gardosi J. Intrauterine growth restriction: new concepts in antenatal surveillance, diagnosis, and management. Am J Obstet Gynecol 2011; 204: 288.

- Gabbe S, Niebyl J, Simpson J. Obstetrics Normal and Problem Pregnancies. 5th ed. New York: Churchill Livingstone; 2007.

- Grivell R, Wong L, Bhatia V. Regimens of fetal surveillance for impaired fetal growth. Cochrane Database Syst Rev. 2012; 6: CD007113.

- Haas D, Imperiale T, Kirkpatrick P, et al. Tocolytic therapy: a meta-analysis and decision analysis. Obstet Gynecol 2009; 113: 585.

- Knee K, Eason E. SOGC Clinical Practice Guidelines. Prevention of Rh Alloimmunization. J Obstet Gynecol Can. 2003; 25: 765.

- Lausman A, McCarthy F, Walker M, et al. Screening, diagnosis, and management of intrauterine growth restriction. J Obstet Gynaecol Can. 2012; 34: 17.

- Maureen P. Danforth's Obstetrics and Gynecology. 9th ed. Medical and Surgical complications of pregnancy. Urinary tract infection. 2003.

- Nakling J, Backe B. Pregnancy risk increases from 41 weeks of gestation. Acta Obstet Gynecol Scand. 2006; 85: 663.

- Newton E. Diagnosis of perinatal TORCH infections. Clinic Obstet Gynecol. 1999; 42: 59.

- Norwitz E, Robinson J, Repke J. Labor and delivery. In: Gabbe SG, Niebyl J, Simpson J, eds. Obstetrics: Normal and problem pregnancies. 3rd ed. New York: Churchill Livingstone; 2003.

- Oxford handbook of Obstetrics and Gynecology. Infection diseases in pregnancy. Syphilis in pregnancy. 2003.

- Tay J, Moore J, Walker J. Clinical review: Ectopic pregnancy. BMJ. 2000; 320: 916.

- Werner E, Savitz D, Janevic T, et al. Mode of delivery and neonatal outcomes in preterm, small-for-gestational-age newborns. Obstet Gynecol 2012; 120: 560.

www.ingramcontent.com/pod-product-compliance
Lightning Source LLC
Chambersburg PA
CBHW071218220526
45468CB00002B/659